Fabio Correia Lima Nepomuceno
Sarah Nunes de Freitas Domiciano
Otília Jurema de Carvalho Neta

Endometriosis

Fabio Correia Lima Nepomuceno
Sarah Nunes de Freitas Domiciano
Otília Jurema de Carvalho Neta

Endometriosis

General anatomic and clinical aspects and their relation with infertility

ScienciaScripts

Imprint

Any brand names and product names mentioned in this book are subject to trademark, brand or patent protection and are trademarks or registered trademarks of their respective holders. The use of brand names, product names, common names, trade names, product descriptions etc. even without a particular marking in this work is in no way to be construed to mean that such names may be regarded as unrestricted in respect of trademark and brand protection legislation and could thus be used by anyone.

Cover image: www.ingimage.com

This book is a translation from the original published under ISBN 978-620-2-80843-9.

Publisher:
Sciencia Scripts
is a trademark of
International Book Market Service Ltd., member of OmniScriptum Publishing Group
17 Meldrum Street, Beau Bassin 71504, Mauritius
Printed at: see last page
ISBN: 978-620-3-51197-0

SARAH NUNES DE FREITAS DOMICIANOOTILIA

JUREMA DE CARVALHO NETAFABIO

CORREIA LIMA NEPOMUCENO

ENDOMETRIOSIS: GENERAL ANATOMICAL AND CLINICAL ASPECTS AND ITSRELATIONSHIP WITH INFERTILITY

JOAO PESSOA

PB

1

SARAH NUNES DE FREITAS DOMICIANO
OTILIA JUREMA DE CARVALHO NETA
FABIO CORREIA LIMA NEPOMUCENO

ENDOMETRIOSIS: GENERAL ANATOMICAL AND CLINICAL ASPECTS
AND ITSRELATIONSHIP
WITH INFERTILITY

JOAO PESSOA

PB

2

SUMMARY

Endometriosis is a pathology in which the endometrium is found outside the uterine cavity. The causes are not yet well established, and it is difficult to diagnose it due to the nonspecificity of the clinical picture. In industrialised countries, it is one of the main causes of gynaecological hospitalisation, and in Brazil, it affects around six million Brazilian women. There are several clinical manifestations, such as dysmenorrhoea, intestinal alterations during the menstrual period, dyspaurenia and dysuria. Women who have endometriosis are more likely to be infertile, so there is a need to rethink the practices that are used for the diagnosis and also the treatment for the disease, and with this, it is important to have the support of family members and professionals, because there are great emotional impacts. The present study was conducted in the format of integrative review of qualitative literature on the topic endometriosis. For this, a bibliographic survey was conducted in the period between January and February 2021, using the following databases: Virtual Health Library (VHL) and United States National Library of Medicine (USNLM).

Keywords: endometriosis, infertility, treatment

ABSTRACT

Endometriosis is a condition in which the endometrium is outside the uterine cavity. The causes are not yet well established, as well as there is a difficulty in diagnosis, because of the non-specificity of the clinical picture. In industrialized countries, it is one of the main causes of gynecological hospitalization, and in Brazil, it affects around six million Brazilian women. There are several clinical manifestations, such as dysmenorrhea, intestinal changes during the menstrual period, dyspaurenia and dysuria. Women with endometriosis are more likely to be infertile, with this, there is a need to rethink the practices that are used for diagnosis and also treatment for the disease, and with this, support from family members and professionals is important, because there are big emotional impacts. The present study was carried out in the format of an integrative review of qualitative literature on the theme of endometriosis. For this purpose, a bibliographic survey was carried out between January and February 2021, using the following databases: Virtual Health Library (VHL) and United States National Library of Medicine (USNLM).

Keywords: endometriosis, infertility, treatment

INTRODUCTION

Endometriosis is a chronic gynecological condition, estrogen-dependent, characterized by the presence of endometrial tissue in extra-uterine sites. Its prevalence ranges from 5 to 15% in women in the reproductive period and around 3% in postmenopausal women (MARQUI, 2014). Endometriosis occurs almost exclusively in women of reproductive age, averaging between 25 and 29 years, and is rare in prepubescent and climacteric women. An increased incidence is observed among women with menstrual cycles lasting 27 days or less. Similarly, bleeding time greater than or equal to seven days and presence of premenstrual spotting is associated with this pathology (CACCIATORI and MEDEIROS, 2015).

Among women under 20 years of age, complaining of chronic pain or dyspareunia, the prevalence of endometriosis is between 47% and 65%. However, the true prevalence in the general population is difficult to determine due to intrinsic limitations of health care systems and diagnostic methods. There are reports of familial tendency towards endometriosis. There are also indications that the prevalence among women of different ethnicities is similar, despite the inability of studies to avoid the presence of confounding variables, such as reproductive patterns, incidence of STDs, access to contraception, among others (CACCIATORI and MEDEIROS, 2015).

Endometriosis is an important cause of pelvic pain and female infertility, leading to physical and mental stress, seriously compromising the quality of life of patients, mainly due to delayed diagnosis. The treatment of endometriosis has been a challenge for health professionals. The treatment is individualized, taking into consideration the symptoms, the sites affected by the disease, the depth of the lesions, and whether or not there is a desire to become pregnant. Firstly, the treatment aims to reduce symptoms, and secondly, to prevent the progression of the disease (BARBOSA and OLIVEIRA, 2015).

According to Crosera et al. (2010), the way endometriosis causes infertility is still uncertain. In the most advanced stage of the disease, "the distortion of the pelvic anatomy, adhesions and tubal occlusion have an obvious causal relationship with infertility". However, most women have minimal and/or moderate endometriosis, without evidence of the problems cited (BARBOSA and OLIVEIRA, 2015).

Endometriosis is an enigmatic and "cruel" disease that deserves attention of health professionals, as well as knowledge of society. Since it is a disease of difficult diagnosis, without cure and that despite not being considered malignant, it causes serious damage to the life of women, extending consequently to their families. It affects not only the physical aspect, but also the psychological, professional and social. Since, depending on its stage and form of presentation, it can leave the woman in a state of prostration due to physical and emotional pain, preventing her from performing her daily activities normally (BARBOSA and OLIVEIRA, 2015). Endometriosis has a considerable economic impact on society as a result of the delay in diagnosis after the onset of symptoms, the expensive medical and surgical treatments and the chronicity of the disease, which can lead to several hospitalizations, and the indirect costs associated with reduced quality of life and work capacity (SPIGOLON, AMARAL and BARRA, 2012).

It can be inferred that there is a need for more studies related to the disease, in order to elucidate the various issues that are still obscure to current medicine. In addition to providing campaigns, on the part of health organizations, to warn about the existence of the disease and its symptoms, in order to produce knowledge and reduce the time of diagnosis that has been considerably long, further aggravating the problem, since endometriosis is a disease of progressive nature (SPIGOLON, AMARAL and BARRA, 2012).

CHAPTER 1 - CONCEPTUAL APPROACHES TO FEMALE ANATOMY AND PHYSIOLOGY

1.1 Morphofunctional analysis of endometriosis

The female genital system is composed of organs that perform the functions of providing the female gametes, of copulation, of fecundation, of receiving, housing and maintaining the developing conceptual product and of expulsion at birth. In addition, the breasts, although belonging to the integumentary system, are attached to this system due to their lactation function to nourish the infant (DANGELO, 2013).

Anatomically and functionally, we have the ovaries which produce the female gametes, or oocytes, at the end of puberty. Besides this gametogenic function, they also produce hormones, such as estrogens and progesterone, which control the development of secondary sexual characters and act on the uterus in the mechanisms of implantation of the fertilized ovocyte and the beginning of embryo development (DANGELO, 2013).

The Fallopian tubes conduct the oocyte, which is released monthly from an ovary during fertilization, from the periovarian peritoneal cavity into the uterine cavity; they are also the usual site of fertilization (MOORE, 2014).

The uterus is a hollow, piriform, muscular organ with thick walls. The embryo and foetus develop in the uterus. The muscular walls adapt to the growth of the foetus and provide the strength for its expulsion during birth. The uterine cavity and the lumen of the vagina together form the birth canal which the foetus passes through at the end of the pregnancy. The wall of the body of the uterus is made up of three layers: the perimetrium - the serosa - made up of mesothelium and connective tissue; the myometrium - the middle layer of smooth muscle - during labour, the contraction of the myometrium is stimulated hormonally at decreasing intervals to dilate the ostium of the cervix and expel the fetus and placenta. During menstruation, myometrial contractions may cause cholera; endometrium - the internal mucous layer - subdivided into a deeper basal layer, adjacent to the myometrium, consisting of connective tissue and the initial portion of the uterine glands, and a functional layer, consisting of the remaining connective tissue of the lamina propria, the end and outlet portions of the glands, and also the superficial epithelium. While the functional layer undergoes intense changes during the menstrual cycles, the basal layer remains almost unchanged. If conception occurs, the blastocyst implants in this layer; if conception does not occur, the inner surface of this layer is eliminated during menstruation (JUNQUEIRA, 2008; MOORE, 2014).

The vagina is the female organ of copulation, receives semen, serves as a drain for menstrual blood and uterine secretions and, during childbirth, the passage of the foetus (DANGELO, 2013).

The external genital organs of women are the pubic mound, the labia majora (which surround the rima of the pudenda) and minora (which surround the vestibule of the vagina) of the pudenda, the clitoris, the bulbs of the vestibule, and the major and minor vestibular glands. The term pudendum includes all of these parts and serves as sensory and erectile tissue for sexual arousal and relapse, to guide the flow of urine and to prevent the entry of foreign material into the genital and urinary systems (MOORE, 2014).

With regard to the female hormonal system, it consists of three hierarchies of hormones: the hypothalamic releasing hormone, gonadotropin-releasing hormone (GnRH); the anterior pituitary sex hormones, follicle-stimulating hormone (FSH) and luteinizing hormone (LH), both of which are secreted in response to the release of GnRH from the hypothalamus; the ovarian hormones, oestrogen and progesterone, which are secreted by the ovaries in response to the two female sex hormones from the anterior pituitary (HALL, 2011).

Every 28 days or so, gonadotropic hormones from the anterior pituitary cause about eight to twelve new follicles to start growing in the ovaries. One of these follicles finally "matures" and ovulates on day 14 of the cycle. During the growth of the follicles, mainly oestrogen is secreted. After ovulation, the secretory cells of the residual follicles develop into the corpus luteum, which secretes large amounts of the major female hormones estrogen and progesterone. After another two weeks the corpus luteum degenerates, at which point the hormones estrogen and progesterone are greatly reduced and menstruation occurs. A new ovarian cycle, then, follows (HALL, 2011).

1.2 Theories on the pathophysiology of endometriosis

Endometriosis is an oestrogen-dependent gynecological disease characterized by the presence of viable endometrial tissue outside the uterine cavity. This tissue is called endometriotic lesion and can be found in the ovaries, peritoneum, uterine tubes, bladder, intestines and other organs (FREITAS, 2013).

In pathological evaluation, endometriosis varies from the presence of microscopic foci to large endometriotic cysts (endometriomas). The smaller implants are red, petechial and may also have a white or yellowish appearance in younger lesions. With subsequent growth and maturation of the lesion, "menstrual" debris accumulates, giving it a chystic, dark brown, dark blue or black appearance. The adjacent peritoneal surface becomes thickened and scarred. The implants may change appearance during the menstrual cycle, becoming swollen and congested during menstruation and in some cases bleeding may occur. As the disease progresses, the number and size of the lesions increase and extensive adherent processes and fibrosis develop. Extensive adhesions may even distort the normal pelvic anatomy, obliterating the Douglas cul-de-sac (CAMPOS et al., 2008).

When present in the ovary, endometriotic cysts can grow to several centimetres (rarely exceeding 15 cm) and are called endometriomas or 'chocolate cysts'. They are the result of repeated cyclical bleeding from a deep implant. They can completely replace normal ovarian tissue. These cysts are usually thick-walled and fibrotic and have areas of discolouration and thick fibrous adhesions. Large lesions or lesions with nodularity of the wall should be carefully evaluated in order to exclude malignant disease (CAMPOS et al., 2008).

Endometriosis is a polygenetic and multifactorial disease, however, its pathophysiological mechanism is not yet fully understood. The mechanism by which the lesions establish themselves outside the uterine cavity and become a functional tissue remains unclear and studies have proposed several theories to explain this development (FREITAS, 2013).

Originally proposed by Sampson in the mid-1920s, the retrograde menstruation theory is based on the assumption that endometriosis is caused by the implantation of endometrial cells by tubal regurgitation during menstruation (CARAQA et al., 2011). Several studies corroborate the retrograde menstruation when compared to non-affected women, in addition, patients with endometriosis have an abnormal myometrial contraction pattern, women with mullerian anomalies and cervical or vaginal obstruction have a higher risk of developing endometriosis early (OLIVEIRA et al., 2010).

The fact that only a fraction of women with retrograde menstruation develop endometriosis suggests the participation of other adjuvant factors. A greater viability of implants, associated with immunological and peritoneal fluid changes, which allow their adhesion, implantation, neovascularisation and survival, are factors possibly involved in the pathogenesis of this disease (OLIVEIRA et al., 2010). This theory is supported by the occurrence of cutaneous endometriosis in scar regions of laparoscopy, such as umbilical endometriosis (CACCIATORI and MEDEIROS, 2015).

The involvement of immunological factors in the pathophysiology of endometriosis is supported by the finding of a higher incidence of autoimmune pathologies in women with endometriosis. These women present immunological alterations such as: a higher amount of activated macrophages, increased proinflammatory cytokines and growth factors, decreased cellular immunity and decreased activity of NK cells. The existence of a retrograde transtubal menstrual flow triggers a local inflammatory reaction associated with the recruitment of activated macrophages and leucocytes. IL-6, secreted by peritoneal macrophages, seems to play a significant role in the development and maintenance of endometriotic implants. In these patients, the theory of the existence of a deficit immune response, which prevents the elimination of menstrual residues and promotes implantation and local growth of endometrial tissue, may complement the implantation theory (VERRAEST, 2018).

The cell metaplasia theory suggests the transformation of the cell epithelium into endometrial tissue. This theory suggests that endometriosis lesions may originate directly from a process of metaplasic differentiation induced by activation of an oncogenic allele (CARAQA et al., 2011). The theory of cell metaplasia becomes attractive because it explains the occurrence of endometriosis at any location in the body or even when it occurs before menarche, besides the rare occurrence in males. It seems to be the most likely pathophysiology in the case of endometriotic cysts, which arise from a metaplasia of the mesothelium invaginap (OLIVEIRA et al., 2010).

The embryonic remnant theory proposes that cells of mullerian origin within the peritoneal cavity could induce the formation of endometrial tissue when subjected to certain stimuli. This could explain the presence of endometriosis in the rectovaginal septum, as well as in locations along the migration pathway of the embryonic mullerian system. As the embryo initially develops specific female embryological structures, which regress with the activation of the male genome, this theory could also justify the rare occurrence of endometriosis in males. This hypothesis remains only speculative, since it would imply the persistence of embryological remains until adulthood (OLIVEIRA et al., 2010).

A more recent proposal suggests that extrauterine stem/progenitor cells originating from bone marrow may differentiate into endometriotic tissue (BURNEY and GIUDICE, 2013). Some researchers have speculated that persistent fetal stem cells in the adult uterus could reconstitute the glandular and stromal epithelium that desquamates with each menstrual cycle. Recent studies also suggest that bone marrow could be an alternative source of endometrial stem cells. This hypothesis is based on the assumption that circulating bone marrow-derived stem cells (BMTSCs) are capable of differentiating into multiple cell types, including endothelial cells, hepatocytes, neurons, skin cells, cardiomyocytes, and gastrointestinal epithelium. Moreover, endometrial ablation techniques present a substantially high failure rate, with the possibility of reconstitution of the normal endometrium (SASSON and TAYLOR, 2008).

Support for theories advocating a non-endometrial origin for endometriosis is derived from clinical reports of histologically confirmed endometriotic tissue in patients without menstrual endometrium, such as individuals with Rokitansky-Kuster-Hauser syndrome and men with prostate cancer undergoing high-dose estrogen treatment (BURNEY and GIUDICE, 2013).

Figure 1 - Hypothesis of stem/progenitor cells in the pathogenesis of endometriosis

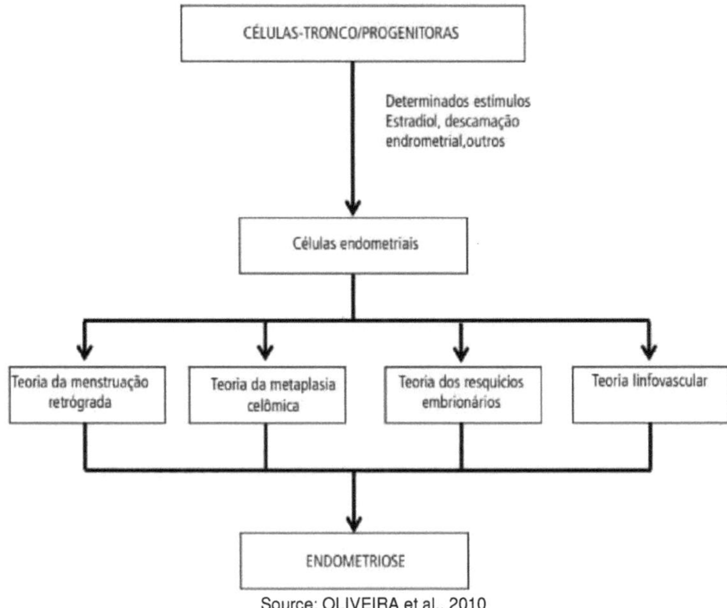

Source: OLIVEIRA et al., 2010

Finally, there is the theory of lymphovascular metastasis, which holds that ectopic endometrial implants are the result of lymphatic or hematogenous spread of endometrial cells. Microvascular studies have demonstrated lymph flow from the uterine body to the ovary, making possible a role for the lymphatic system in the etiology of ovarian endometriosis. Endometriosis within the lymph nodes has been documented in a baboon model of induced endometriosis and in 6-7% of women in lymphadenectomy. The strongest evidence for the theory of benign metastasis is derived from reports of histologically proven endometriotic lesions occurring at sites distant from the uterus to include bone, lung and brain (BURNEY and GIUDICE, 2013).

Other theories involving the participation of environmental, genetic factors and the influence of oxidative stress try to explain why, although a large majority of women present with retrograde menstruation, only a minority develop endometriosis. Recent studies point to the involvement of epigenetic changes, namely the identification of aberrant methylation of some genes (TNFRSF1B, IGSF21 and TP73, for example) in the pathophysiology of endometriosis, being this a dynamic and reversible process, dependent on environmental factors and, therefore, influenced by hormone levels and inflammatory mediators (VERRAEST, 2018).

Perhaps all the proposed mechanisms may act synergistically, both in the genesis and progression of endometriosis, and not only with one of these factors alone. Thus, as there are still many enigmas in the pathophysiology of this disease, research is essential to try to provide data with a better level of scientific evidence (OLIVEIRA et al., 2010).

1.3 Risk factors and their epidemiological indices

Endometriosis is a common gynaecological condition affecting 15% of women in the reproductive period and up to 5% in the postmenopausal phase. Currently there is an annual increase in the incidence of endometriosis due to the wide use of laparoscopy as a diagnostic method, and it is estimated that the number of women with endometriosis is 7 million in the USA and more than 70 million worldwide, and in developed countries, it is one of the main causes of gynecological hospitalization (RAMPINELLI; MILANESE; MADEIRA, 2013).

Regarding the age range, in the studies by Rampinelli, Milanese and Madeira (2013), the mean age of patients at diagnosis was 34.40 years, with the minimum observed being 22 and the maximum 46 years. A similar fact was found in the data from the Ministry of Health, collected from 2010 to 2019 by DataSUS, of 153702 patients 42.6% were in the age range 40-49 years and 23.7% between 30-39 years. Moreover, from 10 years of age onwards, the diagnosis tends to increase in incidence with age, with the first symptoms appearing in early adolescence. The risk of disease in women aged 45-49 years is about three times higher when compared to women aged 15-19 years, probably due to persistent estrogenic hormone action for a long time (SANTOS et al., 2012).

Moreover, since the age group between 20 and 29 years old, there has been a significant increase in the number of cases, which can be explained by the possible ignorance of post-menarcheal menstrual cycles, the idea that menstrual periods are painful, as well as the difficulty in performing gynaecological examinations in younger patients, which generates less information collected for a possible diagnostic suspicion (SALOME et al., 2020).

Figure 2 - Incidence of endometriosis in Brazil according to age group in the years 2010 to 2019

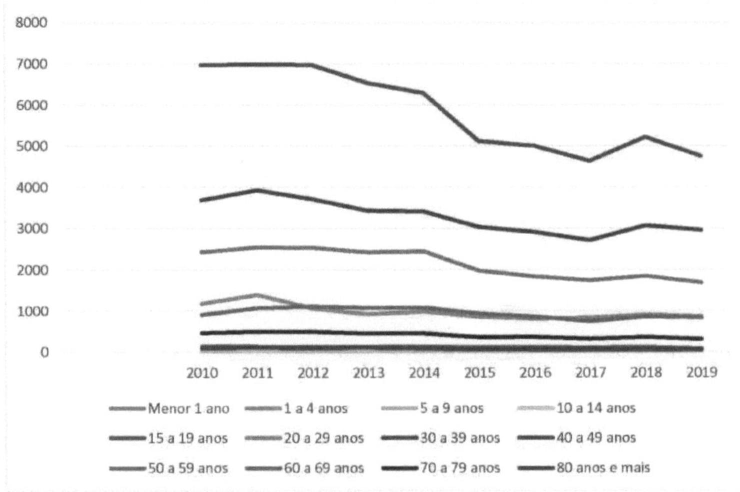

Source: Ministry of Health - SUS Hospital Information System (SIH/SUS)

In the study by Bellelis et al. (2010), a predominance of affected white women was observed. An important difference was also observed between black and yellow races, in which the latter represented only 4.6% of the total number of patients. Data from the Ministry of Health, collected from 2010 to 2019 by DataSUS confirm these data, of 153702 patients about 38.4% were white. It should be remembered that most studies find differences in prevalence between the various races, but these are not statistically significant, which leads to not crediting racial differences between risk factors for the disease (STEFANSSON et al., 2002).

Figure 3 - Incidence of endometriosis in Brazil according to race in the years 2010 to 2019

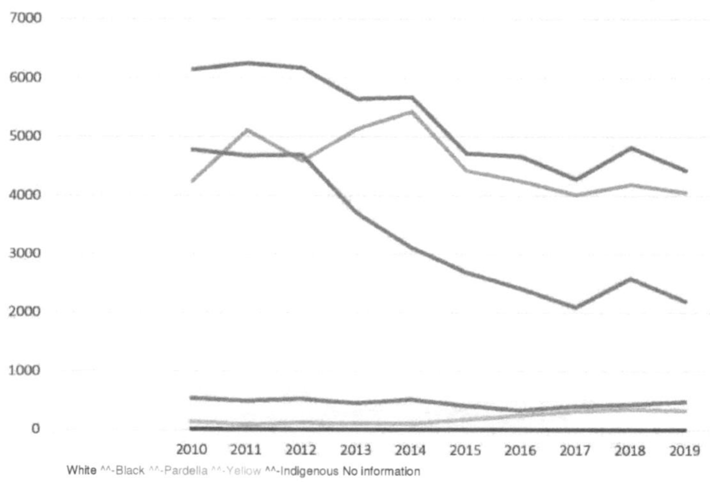

Source: Ministry of Health - SUS Hospital Information System (SIH/SUS)

Regarding the incidence according to the regions of Brazil, the one with more collected cases of endometriosis was the Southeast, of 138641 patients approximately 42.1% belonged to it, while the North region has only 5.7% of cases, according to data from the Ministry of Health, collected from 2010 to 2019 by DataSUS. The population size of the region may help explain the indices found, since according to the Brazilian Institute of Geography and Statistics (IBGE), the Southeast corresponds to approximately 42.04% of the national population. In addition, the Southeastern region has the highest concentration of specialists in gynecology and obstetrics, which also confirms the greater amount of care in this region, while the Northern region has the lowest concentration, explaining the lower number of care (SALOME et al., 2020).

Figure 4 - Incidence of endometriosis in Brazilian regions in the years 2010 to 2019

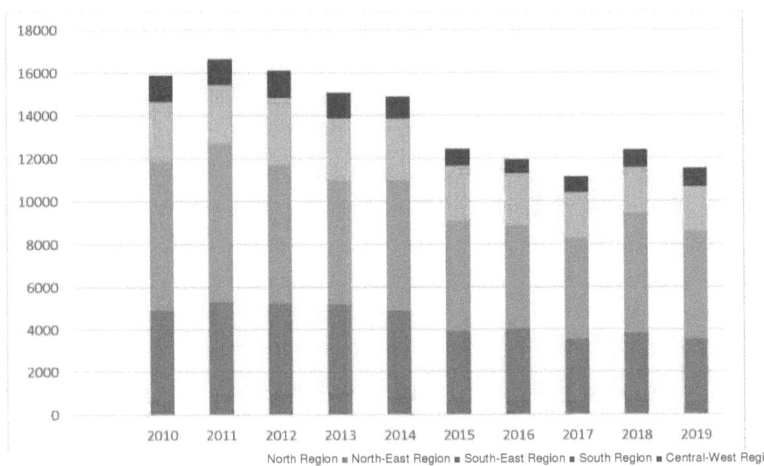

Source: Ministry of Health - SUS Hospital Information System (SIH/SUS)

Regarding the other sociodemographic characteristics, in the study by Silva et al. (2019), most patients were married (55.6%), and the others were single (22.2%) and in a stable union (16.7%). In percentage values, 81.3% of patients had 8 to 11 years of education and the remaining 12 or more years (18.8%). In the study by Bellelis et al. (2010), similar data are found, a

Most patients were also married or in a stable union (69.5%), and most had completed the second or third level of education. The educational level among women with endometriosis tended to be higher, as did the socioeconomic level. This may be due to a bias towards greater access to medical care and greater concern for individual health when dealing with pelvic pain or infertility.

Regarding the presence of previous diseases and risk factors, in the study by Silva et al. (2019) there was an equal relation between them: diabetes mellitus (5.0%), systemic arterial hypertension (5.0%), anxiety (5.0%), depression (5.0%), hepatic steatosis (5.0%), thyroid nodule (5.0%), panic disorder (5.0%), alcohol consumption (5.0%). No history of smoking was found among the patients. Regarding previous abdominal surgeries, there was a greater relapse of caesarean sections (20.0%), diagnostic laparoscopy (15.0%) and umbilical hernioplasty (10%). In the study by Oliveira et al. (2015), it was observed that

17

among the most prevalent diseases under treatment, the prevalence of metabolic diseases stands out (8.4%), which include hypercholesterolemia and hypertriglyceridemia, hyperuricemia, iron-deficiency anemia, *diabetes mellitus* type 1 and 2, arterial hypertension and metabolic syndrome.

The risk of developing endometriotic lesions increases with excessive dietary intake and body mass index (BMI) also appears to have implications. Several studies have shown an inverse relationship of proportionality between BMI and endometriosis: women with endometriosis have often been found to have a lower BMI than healthy women. This relationship, still not understood, may stem from an association between the genetic factors which determine endometriosis and those corresponding to BMI. It is also accepted that low BMI may be due to loss of appetite caused by pelvic pain. If this hypothesis is confirmed, the categorization of BMI as a risk factor for endometriosis will be contested (RIBEIRO, 2016).

Regarding nutritional aspects, studies show that women who consume red meat, fats from animal sources and trans fats had a higher risk of developing endometriosis. On the other hand, the consumption of dairy products, omega-3 fatty acids, fruits and vegetables may be a protective factor, as well as the consumption of some micronutrients, such as thiamine, folate, vitamin C and vitamin E. Regarding symptom control, the restriction of red meat consumption and the intake of antioxidant vitamins and minerals are good strategies for reducing chronic pelvic pain in women with the disease (CHALUB; LEAO; MAYNARD, 2020).

As to environmental factors, the relationship between human exposure to PCBs and the development of hormone-dependent diseases has been the subject of research in several epidemiological studies. Most studies of endometriosis have focused on one form of PCB, dioxin, although no association has been found. Due to the recognized ability of PCBs to alter the endometrial function, both in animals and in humans, one can try to relate the action of these pollutants in the etiopathogenesis of this disease (BELLELIS; PODGAEC; ABRAO, 2014).

The loss of endometrial sensitivity to progesterone is recognised as a potential causative factor in endometriosis. During the menstrual cycle, as progesterone levels decrease in the secretory phase, we notice an increase in proinflammatory cytokines, chemokines and MMPs, preparing the endometrium for the intense inflammatory process of menstruation. Furthermore, PCBs/TCDD + AhR receptor complexes may activate proinflammatory cytokine and chemokine genes, possibly leading to a chronic pattern of pro-inflammatory signaling that would disrupt normal endometrial function. Moreover, the combination of TCDD and estradiol may further enhance this pro-inflammatory effect, increasing the invasion capacity of endometrial stromal cells (BELLELIS; PODGAEC; ABRAO, 2014).

The analysis of family history showed depression (21.1%) as the most frequently reported disease. Few consistent studies associate the presence of endometriosis in family history and other associated diseases, but they conclude that there is a higher risk of having the disease in patients with first-degree relatives with endometriosis (OLIVEIRA et al., 2015).

The genetic influence of endometriosis is complex and remains unexplained. However, most researchers believe that the inheritance is polygenic and multifactorial, i.e. the phenotype is determined by a combination of multiple genes *and* environmental factors. The increased risk of disease in individuals who have affected family members is higher than in the general population. There have been studies showing endometriosis rates of 4.8% to 8.8% in the siblings of endometriosis patients. Several studies have found three to nine times increased risk for sisters and mothers of women with endometriosis, besides studies with twins showing that the concordance between monozygotic twins is twice as high as the concordance between dizygotic twins (BELLELIS et al., 2010; SANTOS et al., 2011).

Moreover, genetic polymorphisms seem to have an influence in the etiology of the disease, helping the adhesion and proliferation of endometrial tissue cells in the peritoneal cavity, and thus helping to maintain the disease. Variations in GSTM1 and CYP1A1 genes expose the cells to more toxicity, as they do not exert their function correctly. MMP 2 and 13 help the invasion of ectopic tissue by degrading the extracellular matrix. The altered EMX2 gene may act in the proliferation of ectopic endometrium, however, no study has correlated polymorphisms in this gene with the disease (SANTOS et al., 2011).

Regarding obstetric history, nulliparity has been consistently portrayed as having a strong association with endometriosis, and up to 25-35% of infertile women have endometriosis, and 30-40% of women with endometriosis are infertile. The mechanism for infertility associated with endometriosis depends in part on the stage of the disease, the anatomical distortion by pelvic and ovarian adhesions and/or the production of substances (cytokines, growth factors, prostaglandins) that end up disrupting normal ovarian function and tubo-ovarian motility. In fact few consistent studies have been conducted to determine whether nulliparity is a risk factor for the disease or if patients with endometriosis have greater difficulty in becoming pregnant (RAMPINELLI; MILANESE; MADEIRA, 2013).

Moreover, since it is an estrogen-dependent disease, an increased risk is observed in conditions that increase exposure to this hormone. Thus, it may be more prevalent in women with early menarche, late menopause, shorter intervals between menstruations and longer duration of the menstrual flow (NYHOLT et al., 2009).

In the studies by Silva et al. (2019), most patients had no pregnancies (45.0%), with the remainder distributed as 1 (35.0%), 2 (10.0%) and 3 (10.0%). Regarding the number of deliveries, the majority was classified as nulliparous (55.0%) and primigravida (35.0%), with the remaining two deliveries (10.0%). Regarding the number of abortions, the majority had no abortion (75.0%) and the others had only one (20.0%) and 2 (5%). Regarding gynaecological characteristics, the age of women during menarche ranged from 10 to 15 years and presented a median of 13.0 years. During the coitus, the age ranged from 15 to 41 years and the median was 18 years. The number of partners ranged from one to eight with a median of two.

Also, certain gestational complications, such as prematurity and intrauterine exposure to diethylstilbestrol, may increase the risk of the fetus developing the disease in adulthood. Breastfeeding seems to have a protective effect for the mother (RIBEIRO, 2016).

Regular consumption of soya beverages during childhood is associated with an increased risk of endometriosis, probably due to its tour of isoflavones structurally identical to oestradiol. Indeed, an animal model study showed that early administration of an isoflavone, genistein, resulted in changes in the uterus and in the hypothalamic-pituitary-ovarian axis. Note that soy beverage intake is also related to the development of uterine leiomyomatosis, which is also a hormone-dependent pathology (UPSON et al., 2015).

This may occur due to the lack of knowledge about menstrual cycles after menarche, the generalised perception that menstrual periods are painful, besides the fact that the gynaecological examination in younger patients is more difficult to perform and less information is gathered for a possible suspicion of the disease, which makes the diagnosis more difficult and delayed (ARRUDA et al., 2003).

Among the symptoms studied, dysmenorrhea is the most prevalent, and is considered a risk marker, since it may be related to strong uterine contractions, which increase the occurrence of retrograde menstruation. However, it is important to make the association between endometriosis and deep dyspareunia, chronic pelvic pain and infertility. With a prevalence of 54.7% of patients, deep dyspareunia is a symptom closely related to endometriosis, and may also indicate the presence of deep-seated disease, probably affecting the retrocervical region or the rectovaginal fascia. Also, with approximately 57% of affected patients, chronic pelvic pain is a very common symptom and difficult to control (BELLELIS et al., 2010; MCLEOD; RETZLOFF, 2010).

Moreover, intestinal disorders are also highly prevalent among women with endometriosis, along with dysmenorrhea and dyspareunia. Intestinal endometriosis can be found in 6% to 30% of women with deep endometriosis and these women are hardly asymptomatic. While urinary abnormalities have a low prevalence, about 4.2% (OLIVEIRA et al., 2015).

Infertility (absence of conception after one year of unprotected intercourse with regular sexual activity) was reported by 28.6% of patients in the studies by Rampinelli, Milanese and Madeira (2013). It is known, however, that certain obstetric antecedents, already mentioned above, may lead to a greater exposure to estrogen, providing more favourable conditions for the onset of this disease. Besides, we may observe an association with other estrogen-dependent diseases, such as uterine leiomyoma or endometrial cancer (HEMMINGS et al., 2004).

The frequent coexistence of ovarian cancer and endometriosis has been reported, demonstrating a close relationship between these diseases. However, endometriosis is a benign disease and is not associated with a general increase in cancer incidence. Moreover, common risk factors may predispose to both diseases, or endometriosis lesions may undergo somatic mutational events and become cancer precursor lesions (SANTOS et al., 2012).

Regarding the surgical staging of patients, in the studies by Oliveira et al. (2015) 30.2% and 33.6% of them presented, respectively, the extremes of severity of the disease, i.e., mild and severe. Therefore, since we are dealing with infertile patients with endometriosis, we did not observe a higher number of infertile women with the most advanced degrees of disease in relation to the mildest. This is an important fact, since patients with severe endometriosis do not have a much higher association with infertility than those with mild endometriosis, contrary to what might be assumed. Thus, having endometriosis, independently of the degree, is the main risk factor for infertility.

Therefore, having a greater knowledge of the etiopathogenesis of endometriosis and the predisposing factors allows us to make a better reflection on it, thus accelerating the achievement of the diagnosis, since, despite its benign nature, it has great importance in the impact on quality of life, causes pelvic pain and is characterized as one of the main causes of human infertility (RIBEIRO, 2016; VIGANO et al., 2004).

1.4 Classification of endometriosis

Endometriosis can be classified into three forms, from the point of view of etiopathogenesis and clinical manifestations: superficial peritoneal endometriosis (SPE), ovarian endometriosis and deep infiltrative endometriosis (PIE). This proposal is based on the hypotheses that explain the development of the disease and its clinical and epidemiological peculiarities (SAMPAIO NETO et al., 2020).

EPS can be classified according to their appearance into early active implants (red, glandular or vesicular), avangados (black, wrinkled) and cicatricial (fibrotic white). Red endometriotic lesions are generally considered the most active form of endometriotic peritoneal disease, as measured by activity parameters such as VEGF (vascular endothelial growth factor), MMP (matrix metalloproteinase) and vascular density (VERRAEST, 2018).

Ovarian endometriosis presents itself in the form of cysts with varied volumes called endometriomas; superficial implants may also occur in the ovaries, resembling those of the peritoneum (SAMPAIO NETO et al., 2020).

PIE affects approximately 20% to 35% of patients with endometriosis. It is defined by the presence of endometrial implants infiltrating structures deeper than 5 mm, usually involving uterosacral ligaments, rectovaginal septum, muscles adjacent to the uterus and/or invading pelvic organs (MARTINHO, 2010). Deep endometriosis lesions are often related to more severe clinical pictures of pain than superficial lesions. It has been demonstrated that these lesions have a higher density of nerve fibers than superficial peritoneal lesions. Thus, this difference may play an important role in pain pathogenesis (CARAQA et al., 2011).

The American Society for Reproductive Medicine (ASRM) has developed and reviewed a classification to allow laparoscopic staging of endometriosis that classifies the disease as minimal (stage I), mild (stage II), moderate (stage III) or severe (stage IV). This type of classification is of limited use for clinical decision making as the stage of disease may not correlate with symptoms of pain, dyspareunia, infertility or risk of recurrence and is not a good predictor of pregnancy after treatment. The value of this system will be in standardising the description of operative findings and perhaps in comparing the outcomes of various therapies (VERRAEST, 2018).

CHAPTER 2 - METHODOLOGICAL ASPECTS OF ENDOMETRIOSIS

This study was conducted as an integrative review of qualitative type on the topic Endometriosis. For this, a bibliographic survey was conducted in the period between January and February 2021, using the following databases: Virtual Health Library (VHL) and United States National Library of Medicine (USNLM). The following descriptors were used: endometriosis, infertility and treatment.

Among the inclusion criteria for the choice of articles were full articles, in the period of the last ten years (2010-2020), in Portuguese and English. The exclusion criteria were papers that, despite contemplating the descriptors of this study did not contain sufficient information about the subject researched.

CHAPTER 3 - THE CLINIC OF ENDOMETRIOSIS AND ITS RELATION WITH INFERTILITY

3.1 Clinical presentation and diagnosis of endometriosis

The first step on the road to definitive diagnosis is not to ignore the first signs and symptoms of the disease, as well as identifying them correctly and correlating them with the suspicion of EDM. They are variable among women, and may be non-existent (asymptomatic women) or of great intensity, leading to disability. The intensity may vary over time, and is not necessarily proportional to the extent of the disease (BENTO and MOREIRA, 2014).

The classic symptoms of endometriosis are progressive dysmenorrhoea, profound dyspareunia, chronic pelvic pain and infertility. However it may have atypical presentations and in some cases may be asymptomatic. The severity of symptoms may not correlate with the extent of the disease (AGUIAR et al., 2016).

Endometriosis-related pain can present as: dysmenorrhoea (most manifested symptom), often intense, continuous or colic-like; dyspareunia, typically deep, and may persist after coitus, when intense and associated with painful catamenial defecation and suggestive of endometriosis of the rectovaginal septum; dysuria; dyskinesia; abdominal or lumbar pain; chronic pelvic pain (AGUIAR et al., 2016).

The pathophysiology of the association between pain and endometriosis is poorly understood. It is believed that chronic inflammation is the main cause, however, many researchers have identified nerve fibres in lesions of the disease bringing a parallel between the density and quality of these fibres with pain. Possible mechanisms causing pelvic pain in endometriosis are chronic local peritoneal inflammation caused by the release of proinflammatory cytokines, prostaglandins, chemokines and other substances by the ectopic implants, deep infiltration with tissue damage, formation of adhesions, fibrotic thickening and accumulation of menstrual blood eliminated in endometriotic implants, resulting in painful traction with physiological tissue movements (CARAQA et al., 2011).

Analysing the systems involved and relating the findings to each other, it is observed that infertility is the symptom that is most associated with depressive states and with the increase in prostaglandins, since these alter tubal motility, the mechanisms of follicular rupture, the function of the corpus luteum and, finally, implantation, increasing the risk of spontaneous abortions (SOUSA et al., 2015).

Another aspect is the compromising of the emotional state of women. Symptoms such as anxiety, anguish, hurry, stress and loss of productivity at work are configured in the studies as being the cause of a vicious cycle that tends to worsen the other symptoms. The depression has generated absences from work and thus economic damage which can be transformed into dismissals, due to the constant discomforts reported (SOUSA et al., 2015).

Figure 5 - Signs, symptoms and some complications related to endometriosis

Sinais e sintomas	Informações
Dismenorreia	É a menstruação dolorosa. Pode ser primária (relacionada ao aumento da produção de prostaglandinas) ou secundária (relacionada a uma doença pélvica ou uterina).
Menorragia	Menstruação anormalmente intensa e prolongada (excessiva, quer em duração, quer em quantidade).
Dispareunia (de profundidade)	Relação sexual dolorosa, com diagnóstico diferencial - dismenorreia primária; doença inflamatória pélvica; síndrome do cólon irritável.
Infertilidade	Incapacidade de conceber uma criança após um ano de relações sexuais regulares sem proteção contra concepção, ou de levar uma gestação a termo.
Dor pélvica crônica (DPC)	Sensação dolorosa em região inferior do abdome ou na pelve, de caráter intermitente ou constante, pelo período mínimo de seis meses, de intensidade incapacitante. Geralmente, mulheres com DPC apresentam alterações emocionais, osteomusculares e de outros tratos. Por isso, a DCP é caracterizada como uma síndrome.
Dor ovulatória	Mittelschmerz (dor média), conhecida também como dor do meio (do ciclo mentrual), é caracterizada pela dor na época da ovulação e está relacionada ao contato de líquido do folículo (que se rompeu) com a cavidade peritoneal. Pode acompanhar dor intensa no baixo ventre, sensação de peso, secreção clara e, eventualmente, sanguínea, durando até 72 horas.
Dor que se irradia para as coxas	É comum, sugerindo implantes mais profundos, localizados em áreas com maior número de terminações nervosas. Acometimento do nervo ciático.
Disfunções urinárias	Localização na bexiga. Micção dolorosa cíclica, por exemplo.
Disfunções intestinais	Localização no intestino. Dor ao evacuar (cíclica) e diarréia cíclica, por exemplo. Constipação pode estar presente, provocada ao se evitar a evacuação decorrente da dor.
Aderências pélvicas	Pela liberação de prostaglandinas, que promovem o aparecimento de aderências, com diferentes graus de distorções anatômicas. Há hemorragia interna (das lesões), degeneração do sangue e tecido desprendido, inflamação das áreas e formação de tecido cicatricial.
Massa pélvica	Por exemplo, massas arroxeadas no fórnice posterior.
Fadiga	Decorrente do processo de adoecimento.
Depressão	Decorrente do processo de adoecimento.
Irritabilidade	Decorrente do processo de adoecimento.
Distúrbio do sono	Decorrente do processo de adoecimento.

The symptoms with the longest delay in diagnosis are related to intestinal endometriosis, which coincidentally presents the lowest prevalence among the symptoms mentioned, causing abdominal pain, constipation, sensation of pressure when evacuating, pain, bleeding or even stenosis and bowel occlusion. This can be explained because in general the symptoms of intestinal endometriosis are also common to other diseases and, an example of this is the difficulty in differentiating the presence of blood in the stool with blood from menstruation (SOUSA et al., 2015).

Urinary tract endometriosis is a rare, non-specific entity that affects approximately 1% of women. There are irritative urinary symptoms, such as dysuria, haematuria and even repeated urinary infections related to this disorder. In severe cases it may evolve silently to renal failure. There is a 13% prevalence of such symptoms, however, only 0.1% of women considered this condition as the main symptom (SOUSA et al., 2015).

Targeted physical examination includes vaginal inspection with the aid of the speculum and bimanual and rectovaginal palpation, as well as abdominal inspection and palpation. An attempt should be made to determine the position, size and mobility of the uterus, as a fixed and/or retroverted uterus may suggest the presence of severe adhesive disease. Several studies have shown that the reliability of the physical examination in the diagnosis of endometriosis is low; however, it is essential in guiding the ancillary tests to be performed, making the diagnostic march faster and more specific. The physical examination during the menstrual period may improve the chances of detecting deep infiltrating nodules and improve the approach to pelvic pain in these women. Thus, the ESHRE EGDG (European Society of Human Reproduction and Embryology Endometriosis Guideline Development Group) recommends physical examination of all patients with suspected endometriosis, except adolescents and/or women who have not had coitus (GPP - good practice point) (LEYLAND et al., 2010; DUNSELMAN et al., 2014).

Definitive diagnosis is only possible with the visualization of the process, through laparoscopy (preferably videolaparoscopy). This is an examination which, by inserting a telescope through an abdominal incision, allows direct visualization of the internal organs.

The peritoneal foci present as typical (black, brown, blue or red cysts with/without fibrosis) or atypical (petechiae, vesicles, plaques, retrapoes, yellow, white or red nodules). Adhesions, peritoneal defects or vascularity changes may be found. A biopsy of the implant tissue is performed to confirm the diagnosis (BENTO and MOREIRA, 2014).

A diagnostic laparoscopy is not invariably necessary prior to initiation of therapy in all patients. The presence of endometriosis may be strongly suspected in cases of severe dysmenorrhoea non-responsive to NSAIDs, associated with changes on physical examination and US. In these situations, diagnostic laparoscopy is not necessary before starting drug therapy. Some authors advocate that before proceeding to an invasive diagnostic method to obtain a definitive diagnosis, as is the case with laparoscopy, medical treatment should be initiated, especially in adolescents and young women. This argument is supported by the fact that, even when peritoneal lesions are found, they may not be the cause of chronic pain and also by the possibility that the pain can be relieved by medical treatment, which is often preferred by patients (DUNSELMAN et al., 2014; LEYLAND et al., 2010).

Diagnostic imaging has provided advances to detect the disease, such as pelvic ultrasound for ovarian diagnosis, in adult patients it is common to find endometriomas, more rarely found in adolescents. Ultrasonography is an excellent method to diagnose endometriosis, being possible to diagnose foci of endometrial cells in early stages (SEPULCRI and AMARAL, 2007).

Another method is transvaginal ultrasonography (TVUS), generally the first imaging test to be requested in patients with history and physical examination suggestive of endometriosis. It has a sensitivity of 94% and a specificity of 98% in the identification of foci of deep endometriosis. If the examination is normal, the patient may not have endometriosis or may have an initial non-infiltrative disease. On the other hand, if the examination is conclusive for ovarian, rectovaginal or rectosigmoid septal, or urinary tract endometriosis, treatment may be indicated without further imaging examinations. Additionally, for the evaluation of endometriomas larger than 2 cm, TVUS is also an efficient method (NACUL and SPRITZER, 2010).

Additionally, the detection of adenomyosis - implantation of endometrial tissue within the myometrium - by TVUS is associated with endometriosis in about 40% of cases. However, the specificity of this test to diagnose adenomyosis reaches 100%, with a sensitivity of only 30% (CACCIATORI and MEDEIROS, 2015).

The sonographic finding of ovarian varices may also suggest endometriosis, since patients with endometriosis present ovarian varices detectable by Doppler more frequently than patients without endometriosis (CACCIATORI and MEDEIROS, 2015).

TVUS for the diagnosis of bladder endometriosis has been reported as an effective method, with a sensitivity of 71.4% and specificity of 100%. Ultrasonography suggestive of bladder or ureteral endometriosis may be complemented with excretory urography, which may show ureteral strictures. Uroressonance may be used as an alternative method to excretory urography to evaluate renal collecting system dilatations (NACUL and SPRITZER, 2010).

Therefore, TVUS is the most used exam for the diagnosis of endometriosis because it is more accessible and cheaper. However, this procedure is not always efficient for the gynecologist to perform a truthful conduct, because ultrasonography has some limitations, since it cannot accurately investigate the pelvic region and the subperitoneal spleen, which hinders the proper diagnosis of endometriosis (SANTOS; EMIDIO; ROVERSI, 2015).

Magnetic resonance imaging identifies lesions in the retrocervical and uterosacral ligaments and in the ureter, ascertaining their extent and infiltration. This examination is considered as an excellent method for the diagnosis of pelvic endometriosis, due to its ability to obtain images in different planes from different parts of the pelvic cavity and for its excellent tissue characterization. However, this test should be used plus ultrasound in cases of suspicion of endometriosis, because this type of pathology can be infiltrated in various locations of the body (SANTOS; EMIDIO; ROVERSI, 2015).

Other exams are rectosigmoidoscopy and cytoscopy, capable of conducting indirect analysis of endometriosis lesions. There is also colposcopy which helps diagnose cervical or vaginal endometriosis and hysterosalpingography which is useful in the analysis of endometriosis, when it indicates terminal striae, peri-tubo-ovarian contrast retenpation, tubal lumen pinnings, atypical ovarian shop, presence of diverticula and polyps, changes in intra-tubar images, changes in tubal folds, any possible situations in endometriosis (SANTOS; MARTINS; BARBOSA, 2013).

The biological laboratory marker most used for the diagnosis and monitoring of endometriosis is CA-125, which is a glycoprotein of epithelial origin that can be found in normal and neoplastic epithelium of endometrial origin, endocervical, uterine tubes and ovarian cancer cells. Its measurement should be taken from the first to the third day of the menstrual cycle. When it is higher than 100 UI ml, endometriosis is characterized as being in advanced stage. However, only with high levels of CA-125 it is not possible to close the diagnosis, since it is also found in other pathologies (CARDOSO et al., 2011). The levels of CA-125 increase during menstruation regardless of the presence of endometriosis. They also increase in patients with more advanced stages of endometriosis, which translates into higher intraoperative blood loss (80 versus 50 mL) and longer surgical time (125 versus 70 min), due to the greater difficulty of the procedure in these cases, when compared to milder disease (CACCIATORI and MEDEIROS, 2015).

Another laboratory test is serum amyloid protein A (SAA), which is defined as a protein of acute inflammatory cycle, which can remain widely in patients with advanced endometriosis, higher elevation is also found during the menstrual period. (SANTOS; MARTINS; BARBOSA, 2013).

However, it is necessary to perform other exams such as videolaparoscopy and ultrasonography, correlating them with the symptoms felt by the woman, so that it is then possible to close the picture of the disease. Unfortunately, there is not yet a specific serum marker for endometriosis. This is the great target of researchers, who are looking for non-invasive methods of diagnosis, which preserve the fertility of the adolescent and are less traumatic. However, no serum marker that is specific only for endometriosis has been discovered yet (CARDOSO et al., 2011).

3.2 Therapeutic approach

There is still no ideal treatment for the disease, but there are recommended therapeutic procedures, which may be medication, surgery or a combination of both. The treatment of endometriosis must be done according to the patient's symptoms, the stage of the disease and the patient's age, aiming to improve the quality of life, reducing the strong pain and eliminating the foci of endometrial cells (AMARAL et al., 2009).

As endometriosis is an oestrogen-dependent pathology, its clinical treatment is based on hormonal manipulation with the intention of producing a pseudogravity, pseudomenopause or cranial anovulation, creating an inappropriate environment for the growth and maintenance of endometriosis implants (BORGES, 2018).

Clinical treatment is recommended for symptomatic patients who do not wish to have children and those who have not achieved pain reduction after surgical treatment. The aim of this treatment is to provide a reduction of the pain caused by endometriosis, as well as to help prevent or prolong the development of the pathology. For pain reduction, non-hormonal anti-inflammatory drugs, analgesics and some complementary clinical treatments such as acupuncture, physical exercises, lifestyle changes, psychological monitoring and physiotherapy may be prescribed (FAGUNDES; BELLELIS; PODGAEC, 2012).

Combined contraceptives (CAs) are considered first-line treatment for endometriosis in women with minimal or mild symptoms, and have the advantage of the possibility of use for prolonged periods, good tolerability and easy administration. Progestogens are effective in the treatment of endometriosis-related pain, with up to 80% improvement in pain scales (BRASIL, 2016).

Ademais, o uso de progesterona apresenta um benefício semelhante aos ACs nos desfechos de dismenorreia, dor pelvica, dispareunia profunda e dor nao menstrual. Medroxyprogesterone acetate is the progestogen most used in our country, causing implant decidualization. Its most common side effect is spotting, and edema, weight gain and depression may also occur (RAZZI et al., 2007).

The anti-mitotic effect of progestins induces the decidualisation of eutopic endometrium as well as endometrium in ectopic location with consequent atrophy of endometriotic lesions. The therapeutic indications of progestins include pain control, reduction of lesion size and reduction of post-surgical recurrences. Dienogest is the most widely studied progestant in the context of endometriosis. It combines the advantages of nortestosterone derivatives with the benefits of progesterone derivatives (CARVALHO et al., 2016).

Oral progestins and *depot* formulations are equivalent to GnRH agonists and CHC in relieving pain associated with endometriosis. The levonorgestrel intrauterine system (SIU-LNG) has emerged as an effective alternative for the medical treatment of endometriosis. The efficacy of the etonogestrel contraceptive implant in

control of endometriosis complaints has been proven but the irregular pattern of bleeding limits its use as an option in the pharmacological approach to endometriosis (WALCH et al., 2009).

The benefits of the use of GnRH analogs in the treatment of endometriosis in relation to the reduction of pain, recurrence of the disease and the return to fertility do not outweigh their adverse effects. Thus, among the various clinical treatments for endometriosis, the use of GnRh analogs is limited to the period of treatment, being recommended 3 to 6 months, not to exceed that time, and the adverse effects similar to those of menopause, vaginal dryness, genitourinary atrophy, increased UTI, dyspareunia, decreased bone mass, among others (LIMA et al., 2017).

Add-back hormone therapy aims to increase adherence to treatment and to allow longer use of GnRH agonists in women with endometriosis. The prescription of hormonal treatment to normalise oestrogen levels aims to reduce adverse effects - bone loss and vasomotor symptoms - without interfering with efficacy. Although the *guidelines* recommend the use of *add-back* therapies, this prescription occurs in only a third of these women. Different hormonal and non-hormonal regimens have been used, including the use of progestatives and estrogens alone, estroprogestatives and tibolone (CARVALHO et al., 2016).

Another drug used is danazol, which is also the drug of choice because it is an androgen that stimulates amenorrhea by inhibiting the luteinizing hormone (LH) peak, inhibiting steroidogenic enzymes and increasing free testosterone. It promotes an improvement in the symptoms presented, generating a positive impact on quality of life. The main adverse effects reported are: weight gain, oedema, reduction in breast size, acne, hirsutism, oily skin and changes in voice tone. The incidence of side effects reaches approximately 85% of patients (COSTA et al., 2018).

Aromatase inhibitors are a group of pharmacological agents that act by inhibiting or inactivating aromatase, an enzyme that catalyses the conversion of androgens into oestrogens. Several studies suggest that P450 aromatase is over-expressed in both eutopic endometrium and endometrioid implants in women with endometriosis. In the prë-menopause, studies show little efficacy of aromatase inhibitors due to increased secretion of gonadotropins by negative *feedback of* hypoestrogen induced by them at the level of the hypothalamus and hypophysis, resulting in ovarian stimulation and increased ovarian estradiol levels. Consequently, the use of aromatase inhibitors in the treatment of endometriosis should occur in association with other treatments with antigonadotrophic action, such as estroprogestins, progestins and/or GnRH agonists, in order to block ovarian and extra-ovarian estrogen production (CARVALHO et al., 2016).

Selective modulators of progesterone receptors (MSRP) also called mesoprogestins or partial agonist-antagonists of progesterone are synthetic substances derived from steroids that, although they are structurally different from endogenous progesterone, have the ability to occupy the same receptors of this hormone. They are able to inhibit the proliferation of the endometrium, induce amenorrhea and reduce the production of prostaglandin in these tissues (BORGES, 2018).

The therapeutic approach to endometriosis varies, depending on the patient's complaint - pelvic pain or infertility, although often these complaints are associated. The most widespread treatments currently are surgery, ovarian suppression therapy or a combination of both. In patients complaining of pelvic pain, empirical treatment with oral contraceptives can be initiated without definitive diagnosis, when clinical evaluation suggests minimal or mild endometriosis. If the patient does not improve in three months, or if deep infiltrative endometriosis is suspected, gonadotropin-releasing hormone (GnRH) analogs, GnRHa, can be used for three months and then maintained with oral contraceptives. If the patient presents recurrence of pain, imaging suggestive of endometrioma greater than 3 cm or suspicion of adhesions, surgery should be indicated (NACUL and SPRITZER, 2010).

As surgical treatment, we have the division into two categories: conservative (preserving the patient's fertility) or radical (leading to hysterectomy). The surgical treatment can be radical, leading to hysterectomy and bilateral salpingo-oophorectomy; whereas the conservative one safeguards the patient's fertility (COSTA et al., 2018).

The surgical procedure ranges from less complex methods, such as the release of velamentous adhesions, cauterisation of superficial foci, to complicated interventions on the ovaries, bladder, bowel, ureters and Douglas pouch, requiring, in some cases, a multidisciplinary team (NACUL and SPRITZER, 2010).

Surgery is an alternative for women who have abundant pain that does not reduce with hormone treatment or who intend to become pregnant soon or in the future (MENDES et al., 2013).

Currently, the use of laparoscopy has demonstrated good efficacy, because it allows excellent observation of the pelvis and destruction of lesions by fulguration, coagulation or vaporization, or exeresis of superficial lesions. However, there is still no evidence as to which technique (laparoscopy or laparotomy) is more efficient in the treatment of pain and endometriosis. Laparoscopy has some advantages, such as shorter postoperative recovery time, less blood loss, less postoperative pain and hospital stay (COSTA et al., 2018).

Women who have this condition with severe manifestations and no desire to have children in the future may have surgery to remove the uterus (hysterectomy) as well as removal of one or two ovaries and the fallopian tubes. One in three women who did not have both ovaries removed during the hysterectomy will show the signs again and will need surgery later to remove them. The objectives of this procedure are: to completely remove the endometrial implants and adhesions of the included organs and to recompose the regular anatomy of the pelvis (BATISTA et al., 2006).

Clinical and surgical treatment can be associated before or after surgery. By using hormonal suppression prior to surgery, a decrease in the size of endometriosis implants is achieved; however, evidence of a decrease in the extent of surgical dissection is unclear (LEBOVIC, 2018).

As for ovarian endometriomas, these do not respond adequately to drug treatment, and surgery is indicated in cases of symptomatic or large endometriomas. Oophorectomy should be reserved for cases of recurrent pain, especially in perimenopausal women. Conservative surgery should be performed in young women or in women who wish to become pregnant. Options for conservative surgery include exeresis of the pseudocapsule, drainage and blunting of the cyst, or puncture and emptying. In these cases, it is recommended to send part of the pseudocapsule for histopathological analysis to confirm the clinical diagnosis and exclude malignancy, which is around 0.7%. Excisional surgery is associated with less recurrence of dysmenorrhoea, dyspareunia and non-menstrual pain than drainage and capsule ablation. Excisional surgery also decreases the recurrence of endometrioma and the need for reintervention, as well as increasing spontaneous pregnancy rates in patients with subfertility. There seems to be a better ovarian follicular response to stimulation with clomiphene citrate and gonadotropins in patients who have undergone excisional surgery. However, there is no evidence on which is the best surgical approach for endometriomas in relation to pregnancy rates after assisted reproductive treatment (NACUL and SPRITZER, 2010).

Intestinal endometriosis lesions are those which infiltrate at least the muscular layer of the intestinal wall. Some details obtained in preoperative imaging examinations are important when planning the surgical treatment of patients with intestinal EPI: multifocality, distance of the lesion from the anal verge, size of the lesion, percentage of intestinal circumference affected and depth of infiltration of the lesion. With these data one can program the intervention on intestinal endometriosis opting for rectal *shaving*, *mucosal skinning,* disc resection or segmental resection. In cases of infiltration of the appendix, it should be removed (KONDO et al., 2012).

Ureteral endometriosis may be extrinsic or intrinsic. Treatment of uterine obstruction due to EPI is initially performed with an attempt at ureterolysis, with or without the insertion of a double-J catheter. In cases of persistent dilatation after ureterolysis, ureteral reimplantation or segmental resection of the affected ureter is required. In cases in which preoperative renal scintigraphy demonstrates non-functioning of the affected kidney, nephrectomy should be performed (KONDO et al., 2012).

Despite the proven efficacy of laparoscopic surgery, the recurrence of disease and pelvic pain after surgery remains a challenge in the approach of these patients. Thus, and because repeated abdominal surgery is associated with increased morbidity rates, there is a need to improve not only therapeutic but also diagnostic techniques in order to reduce recurrence of disease, or prevent the proliferation of non-excised implants (THAN and JEAN, 2017; VLEK et al., 2016).

The standard treatment for chronic pelvic pain associated with endometriosis consists of surgical removal of endometriotic implants, laparoscopically, typically using white light. As documented in several studies, the use of white light has been shown to be ineffective in detecting all lesions, with a positive predictive value of approximately 65% of all excised lesions, varying according to their stage. It was also demonstrated that the lower the stage, the less characteristic the appearance of the lesion was, and the greater the probability that it was not histologically consistent with endometriosis. (BARRUETO et al., 2015; VLEK et al., 2016).

The use of markers for neovascularization, such as *Narrow Band Imaging* (NBI), may be effective in increasing the positive predictive value of the identification of excised lesions. This technique, by using an optical light filter for specific wavelengths, allows changing the colour contrast of the endoscopic image, realpating the neovascularized areas (BARRUETO; AUDLIN, 2008). The use of NBI technique has improved the sensitivity of intraoperative identification of lesions when compared with conventional white light. However, this increase in sensitivity entailed a decrease in specificity, considering that, in the present study, an increase in resepositions of lesions histologically not consistent with endometriosis was observed. It was concluded that the use of NBI alone was not superior to the use of NBI as adjuvant to white light. Thus, the adjuvant use of NBI is useful in the discrimination of suspicious lesions under conventional light, as well as in the identification of new lesions, avoiding unnecessary excisions. (THAN and JEAN, 2017; VLEK et al., 2016).

Another pioneer and promising technique in the laparoscopic diagnosis of endometriotic lesions is *Autofluorescence Imaging* (AFI). This technique is based on the principle of autofluorescence of normal tissues, which refers to the emission of light by tissue fluorophores when excited by light of a low wavelength. Thus, the presence of variations in the intensity and characteristics of the induced autofluorescence in tissues allows the differentiation between healthy and affected areas. Studies have found that the use of the AFI technique is useful in the identification of red and vesicular peritoneal lesions, regardless of their size, and is not useful in the identification of white and brown lesions (VERRAEST, 2018).

The *5-aminolevulinic acid induced fluorescenc* (5-ALA) technique, a second technique based on tissue fluorescence, has been investigated. It is based on oral administration of 5-ALA, which induces smthesis and accumulation of protoporphyrin IX, a strong photosensitizer, in unpigmented endometriotic lesions. When irradiated with a blue light, the lesions stand out, contrasting with the healthy peritoneal tissue. Contrary to the previous technique, an inconvenience of this technique is the need to avoid sunlight for at least 24 hours after the systemic administration of 5-ALA. Besides, it has also been associated to nausea and vomiting in some cases (BUCHWEITZ et al., 2006).

Recently, robotic surgery has been referred to as an alternative to conventional laparoscopic surgery. The main advantages have been the greater availability of instrument articulation, capable of performing movements comparable to a human fist, greater depth perception, as well as the possibility of reducing or eliminating the surgeon's tremor. On the contrary, the disadvantages of this technique include a lower versatility, in general, when compared with the conventional laparoscopic technique, namely the absence of tactile sensitivity, the need for surgical assistance and the higher cost. Thus, in order to justify the use of a more expensive technique, it must show clearly superior advantages compared to the *gold standard* technique (VERRAEST, 2018).

Although the safety and feasibility of the robotic technique is well-established, there are no randomized studies assessing long-term clinical and surgical outcomes after robotic surgery compared with laparoscopic surgery in the treatment of endometriosis, particularly with regard to pain relief, fertility rates and improved quality of life. (BERLANDA et al., 2017; THAN and JEAN, 2017).

3.3 Endometriosis and infertility and the impact on patients' quality of life

According to the American Society for Reproductive Medicine (ASRM) (2019), infertility is characterised as a disease in which there is absence of pregnancy after 12 months of sexual activity and without the use of contraceptives. In practice, with the analysis of reproductive history, the determination of infertility diagnosis is made after 12 months in patients up to 35 years old and after months in patients over 35 years old. For women over 40 years old, the diagnosis is made and the treatment is started immediately (VIERA et al., 2020).

It is estimated that 7 to 15% of couples of reproductive age are affected by infertility, among them, about 6% in women aged 20 to 24 years, 15% between 30 and 34 years and 64% over 40 years. It is also observed a susceptibility to miscarriage with increasing age, reaching rates around 40% in women over 40 years (MEDGRUPO, 2019).

In this sense, studies indicate that 30 to 50% of women with endometriosis have infertility, raising a possible relationship between the diseases. In addition, it is observed that the level of fertility is considerably lower in women with endometriosis when compared to women without the disease (VIERA et al., 2020).

The mechanism by which endometriosis causes infertility is not yet completely known, but several aspects of this association have been studied. Patients with endometriosis have a distorted pelvic anatomy, especially in more advanced stages. Changes in the peritoneal fluid such as increased volume, increased number of activated macrophages, higher concentrations of Interleukin-1 (IL-1), prostaglandins, Tumor Necrosis Factor (TNF) and proteases cause changes in oocyte, sperm, embryo and tubal function. Immunological alterations in the follicular fluid as increased concentrations of B lymphocytes, macrophages, NK cells and inflammatory interleukins have also been studied (SCHMITZ, 2011).

Increased production of reactive oxygen species (ROS) was evidenced in patients with endometriosis and infertility. ROS increase the number of peritoneal adhesions, cause mitochondrial and cellular DNA damage, and possibly alter folliculogenesis and oocyte quality. Furthermore, ROS can cause structural damage to spermatozoa and impair acrosomal repair. The granulosa cells of these patients seem to have their function altered, which also impairs fertility (SCHMITZ, 2011).

Besides immunological alterations involved in the pathogenesis of endometriosis-related infertility, it is known that ovulatory and endocrine abnormalities are involved in this process. The folliculogenesis of these patients is altered, as they present slower follicular growth and smaller dominant follicle size. Ademais, as pacientes com endometriose apresentam diminuipao da reserva ovariana, mas não se sei o quanto disso deve ser atribuido a sequela iatrogenica de cirurgias anteriores. Abnormalities of the luteal phase, decrease in the concentrations of LH during its peak and of progesterone in the second phase can also be found in these patients (SCHMITZ, 2011).

Unfortunately, the approach to the patient with endometriosis and infertility is controversial, however, the clinical picture of the patient, her age, symptoms, time of infertility and presence of other infertility factors should be considered (PODGAEC et al., 2018).

Hormonal drug treatment for ovarian suppression in patients with infertility and endometriosis should not be prescribed, since there is no scientific evidence of any benefit regarding fertility improvement. The only medication that can help improve pregnancy rates are GnRH analogs, when used for up to 3 months, but specifically before in vitro fertilization (IVF) (PODGAEC et al., 2018).

Laparoscopic surgery is considered the gold standard in the treatment of endometriosis associated with infertility. The main objectives of surgery in patients with endometriosis are to completely remove all endometrial implants and adhesions from the involved organs and to re-establish the normal anatomy of the pelvis. Delicate tissue management and meticulous haemostasis are essential to avoid the formation of new adhesions and endometrial foci. Laparoscopic surgery for endometriosis consists of electrocauterization or laser destruction of endometriotic implants and adhesiolysis to improve fertility in cases of minimal and mild endometriosis, and is more effective when compared to diagnostic laparoscopy alone (CROSERA et al., 2010).

The Medically Assisted Procreation (MAS) treatments - intrauterine artificial insemination (IAI) and in vitro fertilization (IVF) - may be indicated in patients with endometriosis and infertility, taking into account the degree of disease, the involvement of the fallopian tubes, age, time of infertility and the presence of other associated factors (SILVA, 2012).

Intrauterine artificial insemination (IAI) consists of inserting semen, with selected spermatozoa, into a woman's uterus using a catheter. According to Tomas and Metello (2019), currently the IAI technique should not be used in women with endometriosis, since it does not prevent the recurrent inflammatory process, and the effectiveness of the technique itself is doubtful for these cases. However, Duccini et al. (2019) claims that for the treatment of minimal or mild endometriosis, the IAI technique is effective, while in cases of patients over 35 years with stage III and IV endometriosis, and with tubal involvement, the IVF technique would be the most appropriate. Moreover, Silva (2012) adds that IAI with ovulation induction is even better in mild and minimal cases of endometriosis, considering that the anatomy of the uterine tubes is preserved.

IVF is the appropriate treatment for cases of moderate to severe endometriosis with tubal involvement and if there is an associated male factor or if previous treatments have failed. In patients with advanced endometriosis, in whom IVF techniques were performed without an associated ovulation induction protocol - using gonadotropin-releasing hormone analogs (GnRHa) - the technique was negative, that is, with a lower success rate. Therefore, the ovarian response to hyperstimulation plays a crucial role in determining the success rate of IVF cycles. In women who develop few follicles despite the use of high doses of gonadotropins, the prognosis is more reserved due to the presence of tubal factors, age, infertility time and the presence of other associated factors (SILVA, 2012; VIEIRA et al., 2020). It was found that there is no worsening of endometriosis after ovarian stimulation for assisted reproduction procedures such as IVF. Therefore, the techniques are beneficial for the treatment of infertility due to endometriosis (CARVALHO et al., 2016).

Surgery performed for the treatment of endometriosis may lead to a reduction in ovarian response, impairing the performance of assisted reproductive techniques. Post-surgical recurrence of endometriosis may also occur, especially in young patients, increasing the risk of failure or loss of ovarian reserve. Therefore, the vitrification cryopreservation technique is indicated, preserving the oocytes according to the age of the woman (VIEIRA et al., 2020). The cryopreservation by vitrification consists in a fast and efficient technique that allows the preservation of the gametes for a future gestation. The process keeps the oocyte structure intact by decreasing the temperature and prevents the formation of ice crystals, which are harmful to the cell (GOMES et al., 2020).

Thus, the adoption of this conduct should be individualized and discussed with the patients, considering other factors potentially determining the success of PMA procedures, such as, for example, a compromised ovarian reserve, as well as on the contrary severe pain symptoms that can be attenuated with preoperative medical treatment and thus, for such patients, improve their quality of life (SILVA, 2012).

One aspect that should be taken into account in this process is the emotional condition of women. Factors such as anxiety, anxiety, depression and stress can aggravate other symptoms that the woman is already experiencing (SOUSA et al., 2015).

In the study by Florentino et al. (2019), a questionnaire on endometriosis symptoms and their consequences on the quality of life of women was applied. Symptoms affecting the patients' personal and sexual life had a greater impact on quality of life (QoL). Quality of life is the individual's perception of his/her position in life, the state he/she is in, his/her behaviors, capacities and his/her satisfaction or dissatisfaction regarding this. The term is linked to health, taking into account the physical, social and psychological ambits (SILVA and MARQUI, 2014). According to this study, dyspareunia is the most responsible for compromising QoL. Another point addressed was the correlation between dyspareunia and dysmenorrhea, reiterating the pain as a negative aspect in the lives of patients and sexual activity, in addition to affecting the reproductive capacity of women with endometriosis.

Chronic pain can lead to frustration, social dysfunction and difficulties at work. Infertility caused by endometriosis, as well as delayed diagnosis, can also lead to frustration and isolation. The negative effects of endometriosis on sexual relationships can disrupt family relationships. Therefore, endometriosis has a serious psychological burden, threatening mental health and psychological interventions should be suggested for patients with psychosocial impairment. It is worth noting that drug and surgical interventions, frustrated or not, and the permanence of painful symptoms are aggravating for the reduction of quality of life (RAMOS; SOEIRO; RIOS, 2018).

The lack of knowledge regarding the disease, diagnosis and treatment on the part of the patients has consequences that directly affect the quality of life of these women, such as: frustration when faced with the innumerable obstacles to be overcome; the illusion of a cure or of conceiving children in the face of a chronic disease that may cause infertility; hostility towards the doctor, since he does not present a definitive solution; in addition to the possible abandonment of treatment, since it is ignored that this is responsible for relieving pain and maintaining the stability of the disease (CUNHA, 2012; ROMAO, 2008).

It is valid to point out that infertility caused by endometriosis affects not only the psychological aspects of the patient, but also of her partners. The procreation of descendants is part of the naturalness of living beings and of western culture. Therefore, people are not psychologically prepared to break the pattern. The lack of understanding and companionship in this situation overloads the marriage and in some cases becomes a reason for divorce (SEKULA, 2010). The difficulty in becoming pregnant can threaten the perception of oneself as a sexual being, since infertility keeps the primitive objective of sexuality out of reach. In patients who believe that having a baby is an essential aspect of being a woman, the self-perception, which since adolescence includes the possibility of giving birth, may collapse. And as a result of this, doubts about what is most deeply wrong with them may be evoked. In general culture, motherhood still remains an important aspect of female identity fulfilment. Social representations of infertility as stigmatizing for women remain powerful today and women themselves may feel guilty and ashamed as if they were breaking a cultural rule (VILA; VANDENBERGHE; SILVEIRA, 2010).

The support of partners, family and friends is important and its absence can lead to emotional disorders. Partners, in many cases, also go through feelings of anxiety, helplessness and a mourning process. The professional must validate these sources of resilience as valuable resources that will help the woman to overcome the difficult phase she is going through. The lack of partner support is particularly worrying when one considers that all patients are going through an uncertain and emotionally charged treatment in an attempt to become pregnant. This suggests that there is a role for the health professional in promoting and stimulating the active participation of the partner (VILA; VANDENBERGHE; SILVEIRA, 2010).

The impact of the diagnosis may evoke the cultural stigma of infertility and the irrational attribution of guilt to the patient for not having prevented the disease. The contemporary tendencies in psychoanalytic theory can subsidize a more adequate psychological accompaniment of infertile women. In any case, the health professional must be prepared for the emotional impact of the diagnosis on the patient and take it into account during the follow-up. Besides, the treatment itself also has negative effects for many women, and some abandon it. Here again, we see the need for a good follow-up, with transparency and human support from the professional. In addition, patients' reports show that the treatment can also represent a positive experience. And this is an aspect of the process that cannot be disqualified by the professional, neglecting the importance of hope, and the size of the emotional investment that the patient makes when starting treatment (VILA; VANDENBERGHE; SILVEIRA, 2010).

Therefore, it is necessary to carry out health aids that favor autonomy, knowledge and empowerment of women about the pathology, as well as strategies that contribute to their quality of life and the minimization of suffering caused by endometriosis symptoms. The literature points out that the lack of knowledge about the disease implies loss of autonomy, brings consequences on decision-making and adherence to the established treatment and highlights the alternative/therapeutic practices (bach flowers, heiki, acupuncture, massage therapy, dance and art therapy) as contributors to improving the quality of life of these women (RODRIGUES; SILVA; SOUZA, 2015).

FINAL CONSIDERATIONS

Endometriosis is an enigmatic disease that deserves attention from health professionals as well as the knowledge of society. It is one of the most frequent diseases in women of reproductive age, being the cause of pelvic pain and infertility. Since it is a disease of difficult diagnosis, it may take years for clinical symptoms to manifest, and even if it is not considered a malignant disease, it causes great damage in the lives of women, not only in the physical aspect, but also in the psychological and social one. There is a difficulty in choosing the adequate treatment for endometriosis, and it is believed to be due to the unspecific or late diagnosis.

The relationship between endometriosis and infertility is still not consensual. Although there are multiple studies showing controversial results, different clinical investigations have shown worse pregnancy rates in women with endometriosis, and even if surgical treatments improve these rates, there is no full restoration of reproductive potential in these women.

Therefore, in view of the above, there is much to be discovered about this disease. Further research on endometriosis should be carried out in order to fill the gaps regarding the discovery of new non-invasive techniques for the diagnosis of the disease, and research that analyses the relationship between endometriosis and infertility, as well as the search for new treatments.

REFERENCES

AGUIAR, A. et al. Endometriosis - national consensus recommendations - clinic and diagnosis. **Acta Obstet Ginecol Port**, v.10, n.2, 2016.

AMARAL. V.F. et al. Development of an experimental model of endometriosis in rats. **Rev do Colegio Bras de Cirurgioes**, v.36, n.3, 2009.

ARRUDA, M.S. et al. Time elapsed from onset of symptoms to diagnosis of endometriosis in a cohort study of Brazilian women. **Hum Reprod**, v.18, n.4, p. 756759, 2003.

BARBOSA, D. A. S; OLIVEIRA, M. A. M. Endometriosis and its impact on female infertility. **Saude e Ciencia em Agao**, Goias, v.1, n. 1, jul./dez., 2015.

BARRUETO, F.F. et al. The use of narrowband imaging for identification of endometriosis. **J Minim Invasive Gynecol**, v.15, n.5, p.636-639, 2008.

BATISTA, A.P.C. et al. **Histological evaluation of the induced endometriosis in rats, after treatment with dexamethasone.** Temuco, v.24, n.4, 2006.

BELLELIS, P. et al. Epidemiological and clinical aspects of pelvic endometriosis - a case series. **Rev Assoc Med Bras**, v.56, n.4, 2010.

BELLELIS, P; PODGAEC, S; ABRAO, M.S. Environmental factors and endometriosis: a point of view. **Rev Bras Ginecol Obstet**, v.36, n.10, 2014.

BENTO, P.A; MOREIRA, M.C. Nao ha silencio que termine: estudo informativo sobre endometriose e seus sinais/sintomas. **Rev de Enfermagem**, v.8, n.2, p. 457-463, 2014.

BERLANDA et al. The role of robotic-assisted laparoscopy for the treatment of endometriosis. **Reprod Biomed Online**, v.35, n.4, p.435-444, 2017.

BRAZIL. Ministry of Health. Gabinete do Ministro. **Portaria n° 879, de 12 de julho de 2016 aprova o Protocolo Clinico e Diretrizes Terapeuticas da Endometriose.** Diario Oficial da Uniao, Brasilia, DF, segao 1, p.53, 2016.

BUCHWEITZ, O. et al. Detection of peritoneal endometriotic lesions by autofluorescence laparoscopy. **Am J Obstet Gynecol**, v.195, n.4, p.949-954, 2006.

BURNEY, R. O.; GIUDICE, C. L. **Pathogenesis and Pathophysiology of Endometriosis.** Feril Steril. v.98, 2013.

CACCIATORI, F.A; MEDEIROS, J.P.F. Endometriosis: a review of the literature. **Rev Iniciagao Cientifica**, v.13, n.1,2015.

CAMPOS, C. et al. Endometriosis - Epidemiology, Pathophysiology and Clinical and Radiological Review. **Acta Radiologica Portuguesa**, v.20, n. 80, p.67-77, 2008.

CARAQA, D.B. et al. **Physiopathological mechanisms of pelvic pain in deep endometriosis.** Diagnostico & Tratamento, São Paulo, v.16, n.2, p. 57-61, 2011.

CARDOSO, E.P.S. et al. Endometriosis in different age groups: current perspectives on diagnosis and treatment of the disease. **Ciencia Et Praxis**, v.4, n.8, 2011.

CARVALHO, M.J. et al. Endometriosis: national consensus recommendations - medical treatment. **Acta Obst and Ginecol Portuguesa**, v.10, n.3, p.257-267, 2016.

CHALUB, J.P; LEAO, N.S.C; MAYNARD, D.C. **An investigation on the nutritional aspects related to endometriosis** - Brasilia: Faculdade de Ciencias da Educagao e

Saude, 2020.

COSTA, A. Treatment of pelvic endometriosis: a systematic review. **Rev Cient Fagoc Saude**, v.3, 2018.

CROSERA, A.M.L.V. et al. Treatment of endometriosis associated with infertility - literature review. **Rev Femina**, v.38, n.5, 2010.

CUNHA, A.C.O. O **direito a informapao em saude do paciente do sistema unico de saude - SUS no Rio Grande do Sul** [research project]. Porto Alegre: FIOCRUZ; 2012.

DANGELO, J.G. **Anatomia humana: sistemica e segmentar**. 3 ed. Sao Paulo: Editora Atheneu, 2013.

DATASUS [internet]. Brasilia (DF) **Ministerio da Saude**; 2017. Available at: http://datasus.gov.br/ Accessed on: 17 Jan 2021.

DUCCINI, E.C. et al. Endometriosis: a cause of human infertility and its treatment. **Cadernos da Medicina - UNIFESO**, v.2, n.2, 2019.

DUNSELMAN, G.A. et al. ESHRE guideline: management of women with endometriosis. **Hum Reprod**, v.29, n.3, p.400-412, 2014.

FAGUNDES, P.Z; BELLELIS, P; PODGAEC, S. **Contraceppao hormonal e sexualidade - endometriose.** Sao Paulo, v.69, n.1,2012.

FLORENTINO, A.V.A. et al. Evaluation of quality of life through the Endometriosis Health Profile (EHP-30) questionnaire before treatment of ovarian endometriosis in Brazilian women. **Rev Bras de Ginecol e Obstet**, v. 41, p. 548, 2019.

FREITAS, C.D.C. **Estudo da via de sinalizapao do nodal no endometrio e na fisiopatologia da endometriose.** Tese (Pos-Graduation in Biological Sciences: Physiology and Pharmacology) - Universidade Federal de Minas Gerais. Belo Horizonte, 2013.

GOMES, L.S. et al. Vitrificagao de oocitos: relato de caso. **Brazilian Journal of Health Review**, v.3, n.3, 2020.

HALL, J.E. **Tratado de Fisiologia Medica**. 12 ed. Rio de Janeiro: Elsevier, 2011.

HEMMINGS, R. et al. Evaluation of risk factors associated with endometriosis. **Fertil Steril**, v.81, p. 1513-1521, 2004.JUNQUEIRA, L.C.U. **Histologia Basica**. 11 ed. Rio de Janeiro: Guanabara Koogan, 2008.

KONDO, W. et al. Deep infiltrative endometriosis: anatomic distribution and surgical treatment. **Rev Bras Ginecol Obstet**, v.34, n.6, 2012.
LEBOVIC, D.I. **Surgical management of pelvic pain** [Internet]. UpToDate; 2018.

LEYLAND, N. et al. Endometriosis: diagnosis and management. **J Obstet Gynaecol Can**, 2010.

LIMA, W.C. et al. The use of GnRH analogue in the treatment of endometriosis. **Rev de Iniciagao Cientifica da Universidade Vale do Rio Verde**, Tres Coragoes, v.7, n.1, p.35-

43, 2017.

MARQUI, A. B. T. Endometriose: do diagnostico ao tratamento. **Rev de Enfermagem e Atengao a Saude**, Minas Gerais, v. 3, n. 2, jul./dez., 2014.

MARTINHO, M.S.L. Role of imaging in the diagnostic evaluation of deep endometriosis. **AOGP**, v.9, n.2, p.1-12, 2010.

MENDES, E.O. et al. Endometriosis. **Rev das Faculdades de Santa Cruz**, v.9, n.1, 2013.

MOORE, K.L. **Anatomia orientada para a clinica**. 7 ed. Rio de Janeiro: Guanabara Koogan, 2014.

MCLEOD, B.S; RETZLOFF, M.G. Epidemiology of endometriosis: An Assessment of Risk Factors. **Clin Obstet Gynecol**, v.53, n.2, p. 389-396, 2010.

MEDGRUP. **Gynecology v.2: abnormal uterine bleeding, endometriosis, myomatosis, adenomyosis, polyps, infertility**. Sao Paulo: Medyn, 2019.

NACUL, A. P; SPRITZER, P. M. Aspectos atuais do diagnostico e tratamento da endometriose. **Rev Bras de Ginecol e Obst**, v.32, n.6, 2010.

NYHOLT, D.R. et al. Common genetic influences underlie comorbidity of migraine and endometriosis. **Genet Epidemiol**, v.33, n.2, p. 105-113, 2009

OLIVEIRA, F.R et al, Celulas - tronco: a resposta para os enigmas da patogenese da endometriose. **Rev Femina**, v.38, n.6, 2010.

OLIVEIRA, R. et al. Epidemiological profile of infertile patients with endometriosis. **Reprodugao & Climaterio, v.**30, n.1, p. 5-10, 2015.

PODGAEC, S. et al. Sao Paulo: Federagao Brasileira das Associagoes de Ginecologia e Obstetricia (FEBRASGO). **Febrasgo Protocol - Gynecology**, n.32 / Comissao Nacional Especializada em Endometriose, 2018.

RAMOS, E.L.A; SOEIRO, V.M.S; RIOS, C.T.F. Women living with endometriosis: perceptions about the disease. **Rev Ciencia & Saude, v.**11, n.3, p.190197, 2018.

RAMPINELLI, H.; MILANESE, B.C; MADEIRA, K. Perfil epidemiologico das pacientes atendidas em um consultorio privado e submetidos a videolaparoscopia para tratamento de endometriose na regiao de Criciuma. **Arq Catarin Med**, v.42, n.2, p.09-14, 2013.

RAZZI, S. et al. Use of a progestogen only preparation containing desogestrel i the treatment of recurrent pelvic pain after conservative surgery for endometriosis. **Eur J Obstet Gynecol Reprod Biol**, v.135, n.2, p.188-190, 2007.

RIBEIRO, D.S. **Etiopathogenesis of endometriosis - state of the art**. Review Article (Integrated Master's Degree in Medicine) - Faculty of Medicine, University of Coimbra, 2016.

RODRIGUES, P.S.C; Silva T.A.S.M; Souza M.M.T. Endometriosis - importance of early diagnosis and nursing action for treatment outcome. **Rev Pro-UniverSUS**, v.6, n.1, p.13-16, 2015.

ROMAO, A.P.M.S. **O impacto da ansiedade e depressao na qualidade de vida de mulheres com dor pelvica cronica** (Dissertation). Ribeirao Preto: USP; 2008.

SALOME, D.G.M. Endometriosis: national epidemiology of the last 5 years. **Rev de Saude**, v.11, n.2, p. 39-43, 2020.

SAMPAIO NETO, L.F. Receptores de progesterona e estradiol e Ki-67 no estroma e no epitelio de endometriose superficial e profunda. **J Bras Patol Med Lab**, v.56, p.16, 2020.

SANTOS, A. B; MARTINS, A. M; BARBOSA, F. J. S. **Endometriosis in its differentiated diagnosis: ultrasonography and magnetic resonance imaging.** Monograph (Bachelor's Degree in Technology in Radiology) - Faculdades Integradas Ipiranga. Belem, 2013.

SANTOS, D.B. et al. **An integrated approach to endometriosis** - Bahia: UFRB, 2012.

SANTOS, L. A; EMIDIO, R; ROVERSI; F. M. **Diagnostico por imagem em endometriose: comparagao entre ressonancia magnetica e ultrassonografia**, 2015.

SANTOS, R.P. Polymorphisms in MMP2, MMP13, CYP1A1, GSTM1 and EMX2 genes and endometriosis. **Rev Femina**, v.39, n.6, 2011.

SASSON, I.E; TAYLOR, H.S. **Stem cells and the pathogenesis of endometriosis.** Ann N Y Acad Sci, P.106-115 2008.

SCHMITZ, C.R. **Estudo dos polimorfismos do gene do hormone luteinizante (LH) em mulheres com endometriose e infertilidade - análise da prevalência genica.** Post-graduation in Medicine: Medical Sciences (Dissertation). Universidade Federal do Rio Grande do Sul, 2011.

SEKULA, V.G. **Impacto do tratamento cirurgico laparoscopico na qualidade de vida de mulheres portadoras de endometriose profunda** (Dissertation). Sao Paulo: Faculdade de Ciencias Medicas da Santa Casa de Sao Paulo; 2010.

SEPULCRI, R. P; perspectives. **Rev Bras de Ginecol e Obst - Femina**, v. 35, n.6, 2007.AMARAL, V. F. Endometriose pelvica em adolescentes: new SILVA, A.D.R.L. **Endometriose e infertilidade: o papel do tratamento cirurgico previo a ciclos de procriagao medicamente assistida.** Mestrado Integrado em Medicina (Review Paper). Universidade do Porto, 2012.

SILVA, E.M. **Analise do perfil clinico e epidemiologico das pacientes com endometriose e infertilidade atendidas no ambulatorio de ginecologia e obstetricia do Instituto de Medicina Integral Professor Fernando Figueira.** Recife, 2019.

SILVA, M.P.C; MARQUI, A.B.T. Quality of life in patients with endometriosis: a review study. **Rev Bras Promog Saude**, v.7, n.3, p.413-421, 2014.

SOUSA, T.R. et al. Prevalence of endometriosis symptoms: systematic review. **CES Med**, v.29, n.2, 2015

SPIGOLON, D. N; AMARAL, V. F; BARRA, C. M. C. M. Endometriosis: economic impact and its perspectives. **Rev Sistematica**, v. 40, n. 3, 2012.

STEFANSSON, H. Genetic factors contribute to the risk of developing endometriosis. **Hum Reprod**, v.17, p. 555-559, 2002

THAN, H. L.M; JEAN. U.K. New developments in surgery for endometriosis and pelvic pain. **Clinical Obstetrics and Gynecology**, v.60, n.2, 2017.

TOMAS, C; METELLO, J.L. Endometriosis and infertility - where are we? **Acta Obst and Ginecol Portuguesa**, v.13, n.4, p.235-241,2019.

UPSON, K. et al. Early-life factors and endometriosis risk. **Fertil Steril**, v.104, n.4, p.964-971,2015.

VERRAEST, X.P.M. **New surgical approaches in the diagnosis and treatment of endometriosis.** Dissertagao (Mestrado Integrado em Medicina) - Universidade do Porto, 2018.

VIERA, G.C.D. et al. Endometriosis: causes, implications and treatment of infertility through assisted reproduction techniques. **Research, Society and Development**, v. 9, n.10, 2020.

VILA, A.C.D; VANDENBERGHE, L; SILVEIRA, N.A.S. A vivencia de infertilidade e endometriose: pontos de atengao para profissionais de saúde. **Psic, Saude & Doengas, v.**11, n.2, 2010.

VLEK, S.L. et al. Laparoscopic Imaging Techniques in Endometriosis Therapy: A Systematic Review. **J Minim Invasive Gynecol**, v.23, n.6, p.886-892, 2016.

WALCH, K. et al. Implanon versus medroxyprogesterone acetate: effects on pain scores in patients with symptomatic endometriosis - a pilot study. **Contraception**, v. 79, p. 29-34, 2009.

Table of Contents

SUMMARY 4

ABSTRACT...5

INTRODUCTION...6

CHAPTER 1 - CONCEPTUAL APPROACHES TO FEMALE ANATOMY AND PHYSIOLOGY 8

CHAPTER 2 - METHODOLOGICAL ASPECTS OF ENDOMETRIOSIS 24

CHAPTER 3 - THE CLINIC OF ENDOMETRIOSIS AND ITS RELATION WITH INFERTILITY 25

FINAL CONSIDERATIONS...43

REFERENCES 44

Table of Contents 49

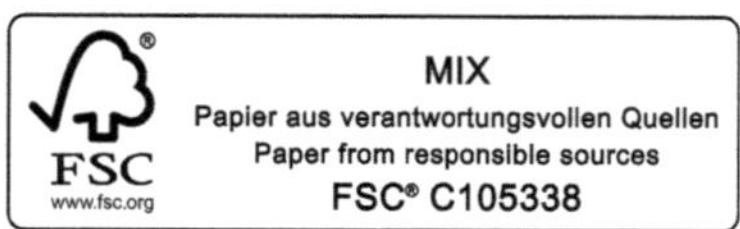

Printed by Books on Demand GmbH, Norderstedt / Germany